CANCER AND MODERN SCIENCE™

SOFT TISSUE SARCOMAS

Current and Emerging Trends in Detection and Treatment

MICHAEL E. NEWMAN

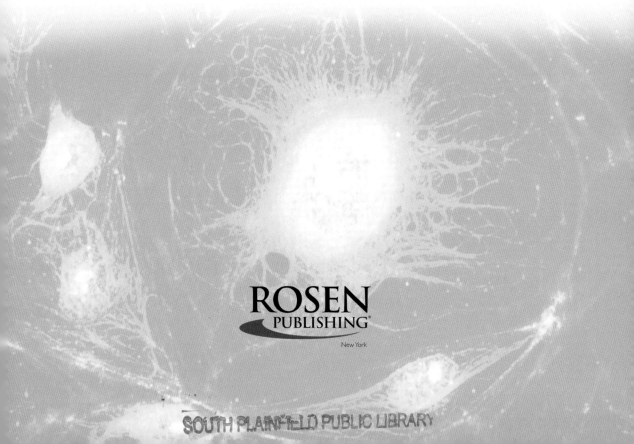

ROSEN
PUBLISHING®

New York

To my wife, Beth, with love for her support during the writing of this book, and to my mother, Elaine, a cancer survivor who inspires others to live beyond the boundaries of disease

Published in 2012 by The Rosen Publishing Group, Inc.
29 East 21st Street, New York, NY 10010

Library of Congress Cataloging-in-Publication Data

Newman, Michael E.
Soft tissue sarcomas: current and emerging trends in detection and treatment / Michael E. Newman.—1st ed.
    p. cm.—(Cancer and modern science)
Includes bibliographical references and index.
ISBN 978-1-4488-1307-0 (library binding)
1. Soft tissue tumors—Juvenile literature. 2. Sarcoma—Juvenile literature. I. Title.
RC280.S66N49 2012
616.99'4—dc22

2010009268

Manufactured in the United States of America

CPSIA Compliance Information: Batch #S11YA: For further information, contact Rosen Publishing, New York, New York, at 1-800-237-9932.

On the cover: A photograph through the microscope shows fibroblast cancer cells being grown in a laboratory culture. The blue area is the nucleus of the cell. Note that the cancer cells have abnormally large nuclei, a trait commonly seen in malignancies.

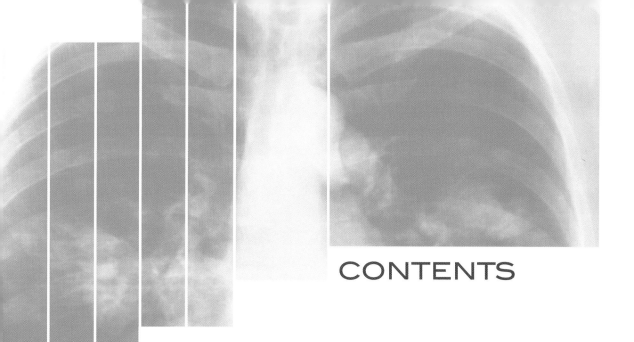

CONTENTS

Soft tissue sarcomas have probably been a scourge to people's health since the beginning of humankind. The first written reference to the disease was in an Egyptian scroll around 1500 BCE. In the scroll, there was a description of "a fatty tumor" with the recommendation that it be treated with a knife. About 1,100 years later, the pioneering Greek physician Hippocrates (about 460–377 BCE) noted that he had seen "superficial and deep-seated tumors in the arm and thigh in older people." Today, soft tissue sarcomas are known to be actually a wide variety of tumors. Despite being rare in occurrence, these tumors can arise in almost any part of the body.

This book was written to help educate others about soft tissue sarcomas. It is hoped that a better understanding of the cancer will make it easier for patients and their loved ones to first deal—and then, ultimately, live—with it. This book starts by explaining what soft tissues are, how cancer can develop in them, and why they occur in the first place. It then describes how soft tissue sarcomas are diagnosed and treated. Finally, it takes a look at some of the state-of-the-art therapies being explored to keep improving a patient's chance of survival and quality of life.

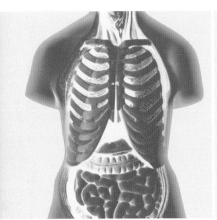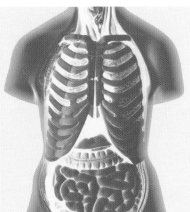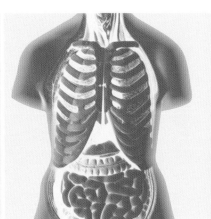

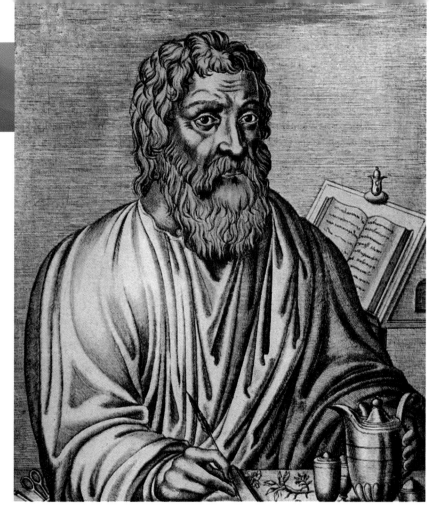

The "father of medicine" Hippocrates described soft tissue sarcomas that he saw in patients in ancient Greece around 400 BCE.

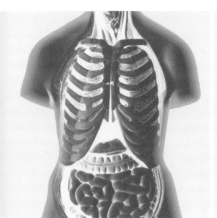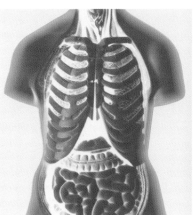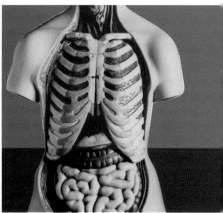

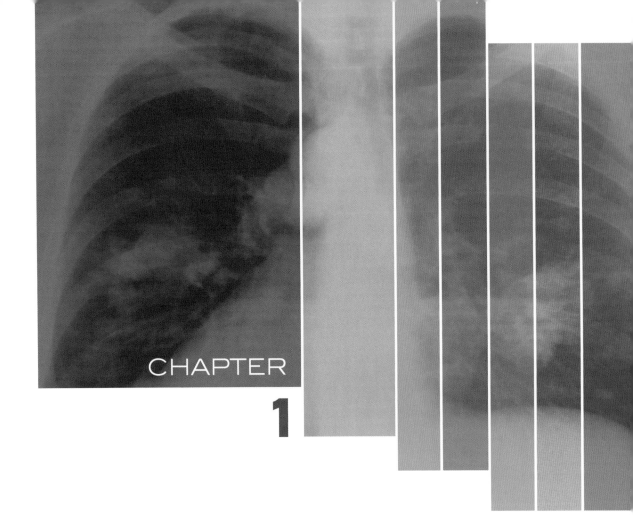

CHAPTER

1

WHAT ARE SOFT TISSUES?

When an architect draws up the plans for a home or building, he or she designs it so that all the components work in harmony to provide a livable, functional environment. Key to any structure's success are the materials that tie its systems together, provide protection, and give it support, such as wiring, cables, pipes, wallboard, plaster, paneling, and insulation. Within the human body, the "materials" that connect, support, and protect structures and organs, keeping people alive and thriving, are known as soft tissues.

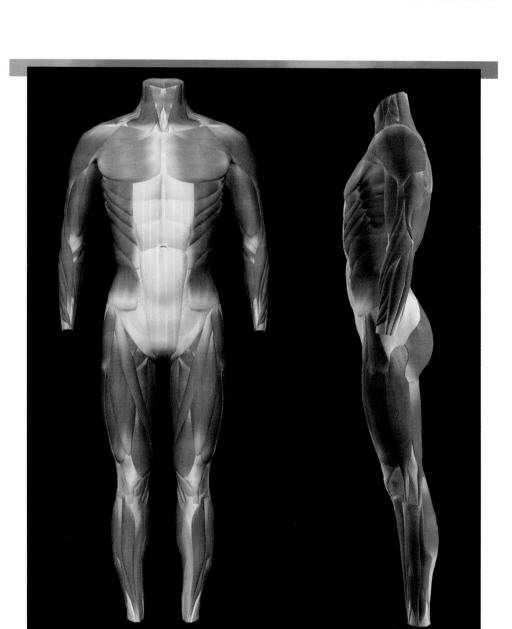

The human body is made up of more than six hundred muscles that allow us to perform functions such as walking, lifting, and even pumping blood throughout the body.

A tissue is a collection of cells that together carry out a specific function within the human body. Think of it as being like a choir with different vocal groupings—sopranos, altos, tenors, and basses—whose individual sounds are blended into a single, harmonious melody. The eight different types of soft tissues are each made up of cells that work as a unit.

The eight types of soft tissues are muscle, tendons, ligaments, synovial tissue, fascia, peripheral nerve sheath tissue, blood and lymphatic vessels, and fat. All of these tissues are discussed below.

MUSCLE

To the fifth-century Romans, the sight of a human's biceps appearing under the skin when flexing and then disappearing when relaxed resembled tiny mice at play. Therefore, they called it and the other tissues like it in the body *musculus*, which means "tiny mouse" in Latin. In reality, the "mice" in people's muscles consist of thousands of long cells called fibers, which slide over and under each other to produce contractions or movements. These contractions support and move the bones in actions that people can control (voluntary). Contractions also occur without people having to think about them (involuntary) in the organs that must work twenty-four hours a day, seven days a week, such as the heart and diaphragm. Humans are outfitted with three types of muscle tissue to carry out these functions. Cardiac muscle is found only in the wall of the heart and works nonstop to keep blood moving throughout the body. Skeletal muscle permits the arms and legs to move. Smooth muscle, an extremely stretchable tissue that lines the walls of the stomach, intestines, bladder, and blood vessels, allows these organs to perform their daily functions.

TENDONS

Tendons are the tough yet flexible bands of fiberlike tissues that connect muscles to bones. When skeletal muscles contract, the tendons associated with them exert pulling forces on the bones to which they are attached. The tendon's job is to relay the force of the muscle to the bone without buckling under the tension of the stretching that occurs. Despite their tremendous strength, tendons can easily become inflamed, torn, or otherwise damaged if overstrained or misused.

LIGAMENTS

When someone who is "double jointed" twists a finger backward in a manner that would have most people screaming in pain, it actually has nothing to do with the number of joints in that digit. These incredibly bendable folks possess ligaments that are unusually flexible. Similar to— and often confused with—tendons, ligaments are the soft tissues that connect bones to other bones. (Recall that tendons connect muscles to bones.) Ligaments keep the human skeleton in proper alignment and prevent joints such as the knee and elbow from moving abnormally. Ligaments also provide a cushioning support to internal organs such as the uterus, bladder, liver, and diaphragm. Like tendons, ligaments may be overstretched or torn. The resulting injury is called a sprain.

BET YOU DIDN'T KNOW:
TEN INTERESTING FACTS ABOUT SOFT TISSUES

1   The oldest soft tissue samples—some blood vessels and connective tissues—were discovered in 2009 within the fossilized leg of an eighty-million-year-old duck-billed dinosaur.

2   Laid end to end, all of the blood vessels in an average human adult would stretch 100,000 miles (160,934 kilometers), nearly a third of the distance to Earth's moon.

3   The study of ligaments is known as *desmology*, from the Greek words meaning "study of string."

4   Sprains refer only to injuries to ligaments; strains are injuries to muscles or tendons.

5   Ankles, knees, and wrists are the body areas most vulnerable to sprains.

6   The overall number of fat cells that people have is set at birth. Obesity is caused by an increase in the size of a person's existing fat cells (which expand when triglycerides are stored in them), not by an increase in quantity.

7   There are more nerve cells in the human brain than there are stars in the Milky Way galaxy.

8   Necrotizing fasciitis is a severe bacterial infection of the fascia in which the invader's toxins and enzymes destroy the soft tissue surrounding muscles. The disease is commonly, but incorrectly, referred to as "flesh-eating bacteria."

9   The fluid produced by synovial tissue to lubricate joints contains oxygen, nitrogen, and carbon dioxide gases. When people crack their knuckles, they stretch the joint capsule containing this fluid. Gas is rapidly released and the bubbles pop, which causes the cracking sound.

10 The Greek physician Hippocrates discovered lymph in 400 BCE, but he mistakenly called it "white blood." The lymphatic system was not properly described until the seventeenth century.

Synovial Tissues

Like the inside of a coat, the thin, loose tissues known as synovial tissues are a special internal lining. They are found in joints with cavities (such as the knee), sheaths protecting tendons (such as those that help fingers and toes flex), and sacs between tendons and bones. Synovial tissue contains cells that secrete a very thick liquid known as synovial fluid. Like motor oil easing the friction between automobile engine parts, synovial fluid serves as a lubricant between the surfaces of joints, tendons, and bones.

Fascia

If synovial tissue is the lubricating oil for the human being, then fascia are the shock absorbers. Fascia make up a continuous web of soft tissue found in all corners of an individual's body—top to bottom, front to back, interior to exterior. They help maintain the integrity of a person's upright form, as well as provide support and protection to all body parts.

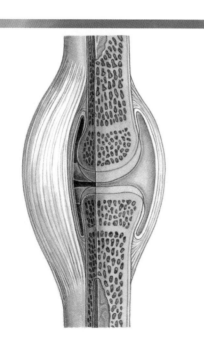

A diagram of a human joint shows synovial membrane (light blue lining) surrounding the joint cavity. Synovial membrane cells produce a lubricating substance called synovial fluid (darker blue).

Peripheral Nerve Sheath Tissue

The nerves of the brain and spinal cord make up the central nervous system, and all of the remaining nerves in the body are considered the peripheral nervous system. The peripheral nerves form a communication network to relay messages back to the "mission control" of the central nervous system. Each of the nerves in the peripheral nervous system is made up of bundles of specialized cells called neurons that relay the electrical signals controlling all of the body's functions. The neuron bundles are bound together by a soft tissue covering called myelin. Known as the myelin sheath, this covering supports, protects, and nourishes the neuron bundles (through blood vessels in the tissue). It also helps speed up communication signals through each neuron.

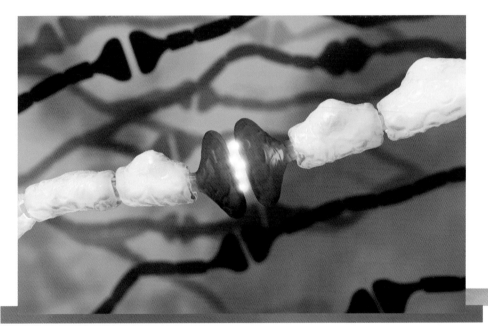

An artist's rendition depicts an electrical impulse jumping from one neuron (nerve cell) to another across the gap known as a synapse. A fatty soft tissue called myelin (yellow) supports, protects, and nourishes the neurons.

Blood and Lymphatic Vessels

In a home, pipes bring water to sinks, showers, and bathtubs. After that water has been used, drains take it away. The two vascular soft tissue systems in the body—the blood and lymphatic vessels—are the pipes and drains that humans need to function and survive. Blood vessels come in three types: arteries, capillaries, and veins. Arteries carry blood away from the heart. Tiny capillaries serve as the portals through which the body's cells get the life-giving oxygen, water, and nutrients transported by blood. Veins are the channels that return blood to the heart from the rest of the body. Although similar in shape to blood vessels, the lymphatic vessels have a different function and generally run parallel to the veins. As the name indicates, their job is to remove lymph. Lymph is the clear liquid in the body's cells and tissues that contains immune cells and helps clear the body of infections.

Fat

Adipose tissue, or fat, is probably the most despised element of the human body. The National Institutes of Health estimates that 40 percent of women and 24 percent of men in the United States at any one time are trying to get rid of unwanted fat. People may not realize that fat tissue plays an important role in establishing and maintaining good health. Adipose tissue consists of fat cells called adipocytes, which are the vaults for the body's energy savings account. Storing the fatty acids called triglycerides is the fat cell's main purpose in life. Triglycerides, in turn, function primarily as energy reserves. Fat cells, and the adipose tissue they form, also insulate the body against heat loss, control what travels in and out of the cells, protect nervous tissue, and help regulate the menstrual cycle in women.

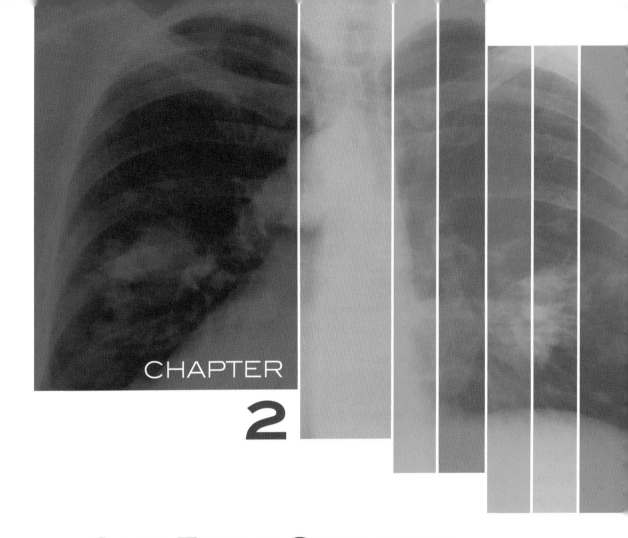

CHAPTER
2

SOFT TISSUE SARCOMAS: A BROAD SPECTRUM OF DISEASES

In 1996, Robert Urich had everything going for him. The "king of television leading roles" (Urich starred in nineteen TV series and miniseries, including *Vega$* and *Spenser: For Hire*), the talented, ruggedly handsome actor had just started a new show, *The Lazarus Man*, playing what he considered the best character of his long career. Offscreen, Urich enjoyed a quiet, private life with his wife of twenty-one years, actress Heather Menzies, and their three children.

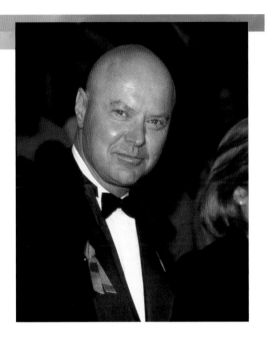

Actor Robert Urich is pictured here at an awards ceremony in Los Angeles, California, in 1997, one year after being diagnosed with synovial tissue sarcoma.

However, things were not so orderly for certain cells deep within Urich's muscular, 6-foot-2-inch (2 meters) frame. Some of the genes that normally regulated the growth, functioning, and replacement of his synovial tissues were now out of control. Instead of producing the fluid needed to keep the surfaces of his joints, tendons, and bones lubricated, the synovial cells influenced by the wayward genes were transforming into unchecked, aggressively growing monsters. Eventually, they formed a solid mass called a tumor that continued to get larger.

When a lump appeared near one of Urich's knees, it was the tumor finally making itself known. This led Urich to see doctors, who soon determined the cause of the problem: it was cancer, specifically a rare form called synovial tissue sarcoma.

Up until his death in 2002 from the disease—one of the cancers in the group known as soft tissue sarcomas—Urich continued to act, openly discussed his illness in lectures and on talk shows to raise cancer awareness, and championed research funding. "Cancer cannot destroy hope," he said.

What Are Soft Tissue Sarcomas?

According to the National Cancer Institute, soft tissue sarcomas like the type that challenged Robert Urich are "malignant (cancerous) tumors that develop in tissues which connect, support, or surround other structures and organs of the body." Soft tissue sarcomas are grouped together because these particular cancer cells arise from similar supporting tissues in the body, share certain characteristics when examined under a microscope, produce similar symptoms, and are usually treated with comparable methods. Although they can occur in any of the soft tissues described in chapter 1, these cancers are not common; about eleven thousand cases are diagnosed each year and represent about 1 percent of all cancers in the United States. Most soft tissue sarcomas, 43 percent, start out in the arms and legs.

Soft tissue sarcomas are named for the body tissues in which they start. The names are often derived from Greek or Latin words describing those regions. For example, rhabdomyosarcoma, a cancer found in the striated (striped in appearance) muscle attached to the bones, comes from the Greek words *rhabdos*, meaning "stick" (the muscle fibers look like rods); *myo*, meaning "muscle"; *sarx*, meaning "flesh"; and *oma*, meaning "to grow morbidly, to swell."

Among the other soft tissue sarcomas and the body areas they impact are the following:

— Dermatofibrosarcoma: Tissue beneath the skin.
— Fibrosarcoma: Fibrous tissues in the arms, legs, or trunk.
— Hemangiosarcoma: Walls of blood vessels.
— Kaposi's sarcoma (named after the man who first identified the cancer): Derived from blood vessels, this malignancy often affects persons whose immune systems are weakened, such as patients with acquired immunodeficiency syndrome (AIDS).

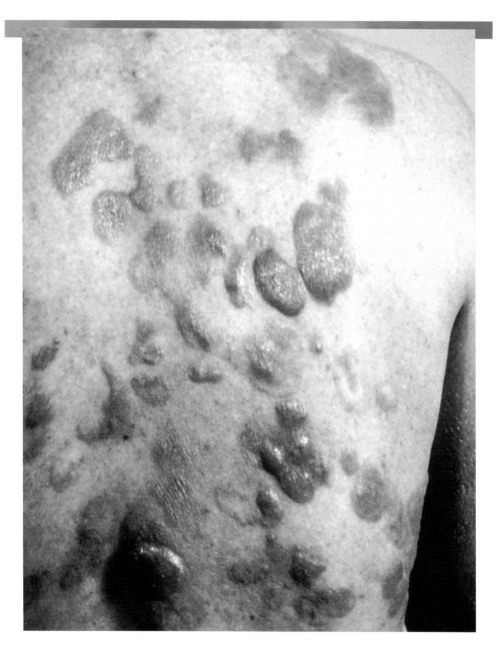

This person has Kaposi's sarcoma tumors on his back. Kaposi's sarcoma is the only soft tissue sarcoma for which a cause—a virus—has been identified.

- Leiomyosarcoma: Smooth muscle, such as that of the uterus.
- Liposarcomas: Fatty tissues, most often in the legs or trunk.
- Lymphangiosarcoma: Walls of lymphatic vessels.
- Malignant fibrous histiocytoma: Fibrous tissue commonly seen in the legs.
- Malignant peripheral nerve sheath tumor: Tissues encasing peripheral nerves.
- Synovial tissue sarcoma: Fluid-filled tissues surrounding joints, tendons, and bones.

Two other cancers commonly seen in children and young adults have "sarcoma" in their names but are not soft tissue sarcomas. Osteosarcoma and Ewing sarcoma are classified as bone tumors.

In all, there are more than fifty different kinds of soft tissue sarcomas. They occur most often in children and young adults, accounting for about 7 percent of all childhood cancers. Skeletal muscle (rhabdomyosarcoma) is the most common soft tissue sarcoma diagnosed in children. In adults, the soft tissue sarcomas seen most frequently are smooth muscle (leiomyosarcoma), fibrous fascia (malignant fibrous histiocytoma), and fat (liposarcoma).

WHY DO PEOPLE GET SOFT TISSUE SARCOMAS?

Doctors know the villain behind only one soft tissue sarcoma, Kaposi's sarcoma—a virus called human herpesvirus-8 that was discovered in 1994 from a tumor in an AIDS patient. For all of the other types, no one can say for certain what causes genes in the soft tissues to change, malfunction, and turn normal cells into malignant ones. Development of cancer surely involved multiple genes being mutated (changed) over time. However, researchers have identified three factors that increase the likelihood of a person developing a soft tissue sarcoma.

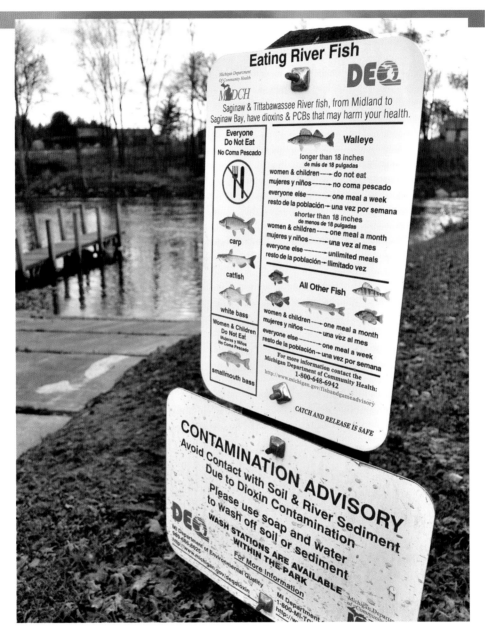

Signs alongside a Michigan river warn of contamination by dioxin. Exposure to the chemical may increase the risk of developing soft tissue sarcomas.

There's an old saying that goes, "You can pick your friends, but you can't choose your family." This applies to the first risk factor for soft tissue sarcomas, genetics. Each person inherits one half of his or her genetic makeup from the mother and the other half from the father. This creates a set of coded instructions that control every function in that individual's body. When the message has bits of data out of order, is switched with parts of another code, or is missing entirely, a mutated gene occurs. If this gene is passed from parent to child, it may create conditions suitable for tumor growth.

That's what researchers suspect may be happening with some soft tissue sarcomas. In one case, an inherited mutation in a gene called *TP53* that regulates the growth and division of cells can result in a disorder known as Li-Fraumeni syndrome. Persons with Li-Fraumeni syndrome have been shown to have a significantly greater chance of developing many types of cancers, including soft tissue sarcomas. Other genetic defects such as Gardner syndrome, Werner syndrome, and neurofibro-matosis also have been linked to increased tumor risk.

Another factor that can lead to soft tissue sarcomas is radiation exposure. In the past, persons receiving radiation treatment for other cancers, such as breast cancer or lymphoma, developed soft tissue tumors as an unfortunate side effect. However, today's more sophisti-cated methods for precisely delivering radiation therapy in smaller, more effective doses have made this problem less likely. An extreme example of radiation-related sarcomas is the increased incidence of such tumors that occur in people exposed to nuclear disasters, such as Hiroshima and Chernobyl.

The third and final identified risk factor for soft tissue sarcomas is exposure to certain chemicals. Vinyl chloride, used in the manufacture of plastics; dioxin, a product of burning chemical waste; insect sprays containing phenoxyacetic acid; and wood preservatives with chlorophe-nols are all on the danger list.

MYTHS AND FACTS

MYTH A lump or bump showing up on a limb, in the neck, or other body region with soft tissue is almost always a sign of cancer.

FACT Soft tissue sarcomas are rare, especially in children and teens. Most lumps and bumps found in soft tissue are the result of injuries or medical conditions other than cancer. However, any lump, bump, or mass that appears should be examined by a physician to rule out the possibility that it is a malignant tumor. Some tumors are benign, which means not cancerous.

MYTH A soft tissue sarcoma in an arm or leg must be treated by amputating the affected limb.

FACT In the past, amputation was a common treatment for soft tissue sarcomas in an arm or leg. Today, advanced surgical techniques—combined with chemotherapy and radiation—make limb-sparing treatment the norm, rather than the exception, for some tumors.

MYTH Children with soft tissue sarcomas can be treated in the same manner as adults because the cancers are the same.

FACT Treatment for a child or young adult with soft tissue sarcoma requires special considerations. Therefore, the treatment plan should be overseen by a pediatric oncologist, a physician who specializes in cancers for this age group. A pediatric oncologist will determine the best treatment plan based on the type of tumor, and this plan will include a combination of chemotherapy, surgery, and/or radiation therapy.

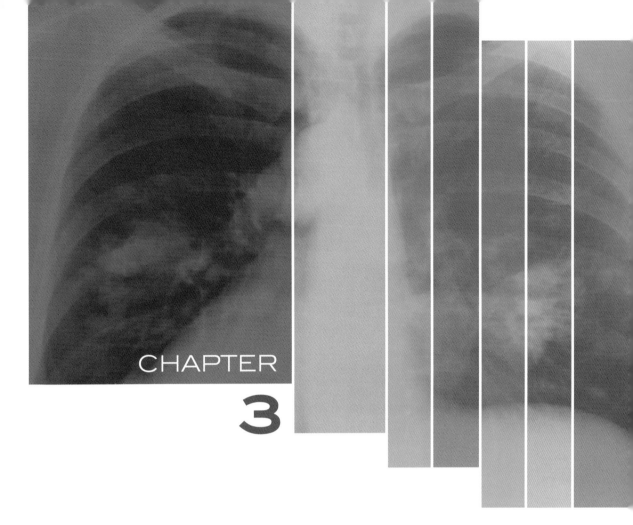

DETECTING AND DEFINING A SOFT TISSUE SARCOMA

In their beginning stages, soft tissue sarcomas are nearly impossible to detect because the patient typically does not have any noticeable symptoms. Many soft tissues are extremely elastic, which may make an early diagnosis even more difficult. Elasticity allows a growing tumor to push aside normal tissue and remain hidden until at a later stage of the disease, when it becomes a large mass. Some soft tissue sarcomas occur deep within the body, too, so they can escape detection until they are very large and cause symptoms.

Feeling a lump is often the first time a person becomes aware of a tumor growing near the skin surface. However, he or she may consider the swelling as the result of an injury, treating it as such or ignoring it altogether. Enlarging tumors can press against nearby nerves and muscles, producing frequent pain or soreness. If the tumor is internal—for example, in the abdomen—even pain may not raise concern because it can be incorrectly blamed on other sources, such as indigestion, menstrual cramps, or constipation.

TIME TO SEE THE DOCTOR

A noticeable lump or swelling that does not disappear after a few days, especially one accompanied by pain, should be examined by the family physician as soon as possible. If he or she suspects a soft tissue sarcoma, the patient is typically referred for evaluation by an oncologist, someone who specializes in the diagnosis and treatment of cancer.

BEGIN WITH A BIOPSY

The primary method for diagnosing a soft tissue sarcoma is the biopsy. During this procedure, the doctor will extract a piece of the suspect tumor for analysis in one of four ways:

- **Fine needle aspiration biopsy:** Tissue is removed using a thin needle. This type of biopsy can usually be done with the patient awake.
- **Core biopsy:** A wider needle is used to get a larger sample from the center of the mass. Patients may be awake or placed under general anesthesia for this procedure.
- **Incisional biopsy:** A small surgical cut is required to secure a part of a lump when the suspect tumor is beyond the reach of a needle. Patients usually require general anesthesia for this procedure.

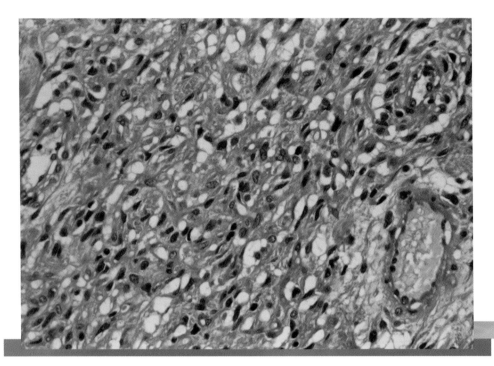

This photograph, which was taken through a microscope, shows a cancerous fatty tissue known as liposarcoma.

— **Excisional biopsy:** A more extensive surgery to remove an entire mass or area of tissue that doesn't look normal. An excisional biopsy may be used to completely remove small tumors that are near the surface of the skin even before a formal diagnosis is made. Patients usually require general anesthesia for this procedure.

Once the biopsy sample is obtained, a pathologist views the tissue under a microscope to determine if the cells are malignant. If the cells look malignant, the tumor must be "staged" to establish the size and location of the possibly cancerous tumor. It is especially important to know if the tumor has metastasized, or spread to other parts of the body.

THINGS TO DO BEFORE YOU SEE THE DOCTOR

Before visiting a doctor, it is recommended that you take the following steps:

—— Write down all of the symptoms you have been experiencing, including details about type, date of onset, frequency, and severity.
—— Document any cases of cancer, past and present, in your immediate family (grandparents, parents, and siblings).
—— Make a list of all medications, including nonprescription vitamins and supplements, which you are taking.
—— Ask a family member or friend to go with you for support and to help you remember everything you want to discuss.
—— Write down specific questions to ask your doctor. (See "Ten Great Questions to Ask Your Doctor.")

GETTING TO KNOW THE TUMOR BETTER

A diagnosis of a soft tissue sarcoma is usually followed by an extensive series of tests and examinations so that the patient's medical team can better understand the status and logistics of the tumor. These can include the following:

—— **Traditional X-rays:** Creating a film image of what's inside the body, X-rays can reveal the tumor's dimensions and help pinpoint its location.
—— **Computed tomography (CT) scans:** Using special X-ray equipment to obtain three-dimensional pictures, CT scans (also known

as computed axial tomography, or CAT, scans) can determine if a tumor is reachable by surgery and look for spreading of the cancer to the lungs or abdomen. A dye may be injected and/or swallowed to make organs and tissues stand out in the images.

— **Magnetic resonance imaging (MRI):** Links a powerful magnet, radio waves, and a computer to create a series of detailed internal views of the body. MRIs help locate tumors and any sites of spreading, map the extent of tumor growth, and can be used following the completion of therapy to monitor for any return of the cancer.

— **Positron emission tomography (PET) scans:** Similar to thermal scans used to detect the heat given off by a person or object, PET scans can produce a three-dimensional image of certain atomic particles (positrons) given off by a radioactive sugar solution ingested by the patient before testing. Some malignancies light up as "hot spots" in the image because rapidly growing cells will feast on the sugar more quickly than normal cells. PET scans can be useful in detecting metastasis. Things besides cancer, such as significant infections or areas after surgery, can also look "bright" on a PET scan.

— **Blood tests:** Examination of blood drawn from a patient gives the physician insight into the patient's overall body chemistry and immune system status. It also helps detect circulating proteins that may increase in number where cancers originate or have metastasized. Blood tests can also be used to screen for genetic mutations that may contribute to cancer syndromes like Li-Fraumeni.

Once the first set of tests and examinations is concluded, the patient's medical team will likely call for further diagnostic procedures to confirm or disprove the initial findings.

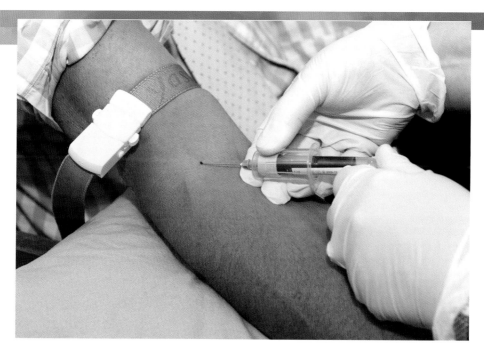

Blood tests can provide valuable information about a patient's cancer that can be used in planning effective treatments.

Classifying a Soft Tissue Sarcoma

When data from all of the tests and examinations are evaluated, the patient's medical team will work together to stage the soft tissue sarcoma. Staging for some types of sarcomas is by the TNM system of the American Joint Committee on Cancer as to its size and depth, designated by the T; whether or not it has spread to the lymph nodes, designated by the N; and if it has metastasized to distant organs and tissues, designated by the M. A grade, designated by the letter G, also is assigned based on how abnormal the cells look under the microscope. The TNM staging and the G grading designations are then subdivided to make the classifications even more specific, as follows:

— **Tumor size (T):** TI if 5 centimeters (2 in.) or less across; T2 if greater. (Note: TI and T2 also may be subdivided in "a" and "b" categories if the tumor is near the surface or buried deep.)

— **Lymph node involvement (N):** N0 if no spread to nearby lymph nodes, and NI if spread has occurred.

— **Metastasis (M):** M0 if no spread to distant organs, and MI if spread has occurred.

— **Grade (G):** A value of X is assigned if a grading cannot be done because of insufficient data. Otherwise, a value of G1, G2, or G3 indicates the increasing abnormality of the cells in the tumor.

The staging that results from the way the TNM staging and G grading labels are combined describes the tumor as precisely as if it had a résumé. For example, Stage IA reads as TI, N0, M0, and G1 or GX, corresponding to no larger than 5 centimeters (2 in), no lymph node involvement, no metastasis, and little cell abnormality. This is more likely to be a treatable cancer.

As the number of the stage increases, so does the seriousness of the cancer. The other stages are the following:

— **Stage IB:** T2, N0, M0, G1, or GX

— **Stage IIA:** TI, N0, M0, G2, or G3

— **Stage IIB:** T2, N0, M0, or G2

— **Stage III:** Either T2, N0, M0, G3, or any T, NI, M0, any G

— **Stage IV:** Any T, any N, MI, any G

Staging helps the oncologist determine the extent of tumor involvement so that he or she can plan the most effective treatment program to combat the tumor. It is also essential to know exactly how big is a sarcoma and if there are any sites of metastasis so that a patient's response to therapy can be measured accurately.

TEN GREAT QUESTIONS TO ASK YOUR DOCTOR

1. Do I have cancer, or are there other possible causes for the symptoms?

2. What kinds of tests will confirm the diagnosis?

3. If I have cancer, at what stage is it and has it spread to other parts of the body?

4. Will surgery alone eliminate the cancer, or will a combination of treatments be needed?

5. What are the risks and side effects of the recommended treatment?

6. Are there any dietary or activity restrictions that I will need to follow?

7. How will my cancer and treatments affect my family members on a daily basis?

8. How likely is the cancer to return after I complete treatment?

9. If the cancer returns, what are my options? Are there clinical trials that might provide cutting-edge drugs or therapies not available for current cancer treatments?

10. Can you recommend sources of information about my cancer and treatment options? Are there support groups for patients with my specific cancer?

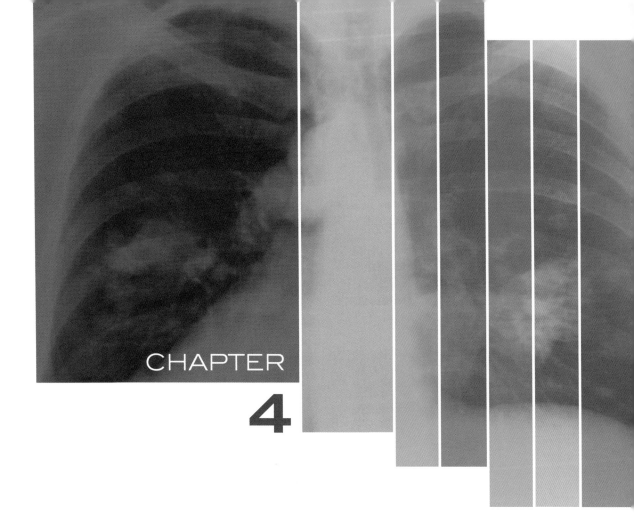

WEAPONS IN THE WAR ON SOFT TISSUE SARCOMAS

As with all cancers, treatment options for soft tissue sarcomas depend on the size, type, location, and stage of the tumor, including whether or not it has spread to the lymph nodes or other parts of the body. The arsenal available to the oncologist generally includes three formidable weapons: surgery, radiation therapy, and chemotherapy.

WEEDING THE GARDEN

Cancer cells can be compared to weeds because they operate in similar ways. Weeds serve no purpose except ensuring their own survival,

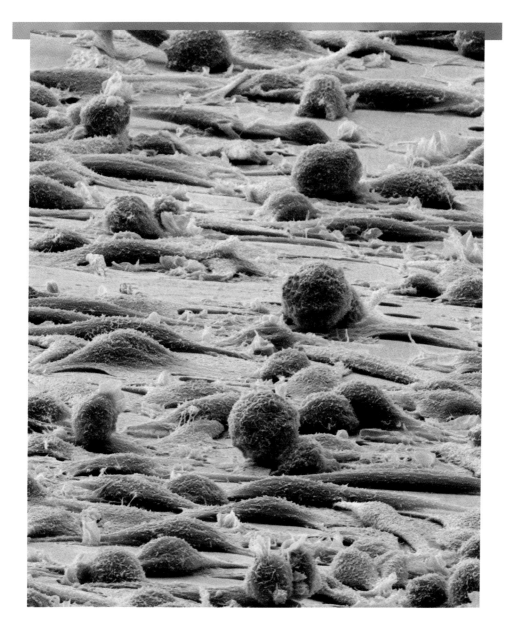

This photograph, taken by an electron microscope, shows sarcoma cells being grown in a laboratory. Researchers study the cells so that they can learn more about them and improve methods of treatment.

and they steal vital nutrients from other plants. Cancer cells provide no useful function while robbing blood and nutrients from other tissues and organs. Weeds take over a lawn or garden and choke the life from the resident grasses and flowers. Cancer cells can spread outward like an invasion force and leave no room for normal cells to exist.

What works for the gardener also is good for the doctor. The best way to treat cancer is to remove it completely.

Surgery is the most common treatment for adult and childhood soft tissue sarcomas. It may be used alone or in combination with chemotherapy and/or radiation therapy. It's important to remove the tumor with a small rim of normal tissue around it whenever possible to make sure that nothing is left behind. For lower stage sarcomas, a simple removal of the tumor may be all that is needed to end the problem. For higher grade tumors (meaning that the cells look more disorganized under the microscope) and larger tumors, chemotherapy may be given first to try to shrink the tumor before surgery. Chemotherapy and/or radiation therapy may also be given after surgery to treat

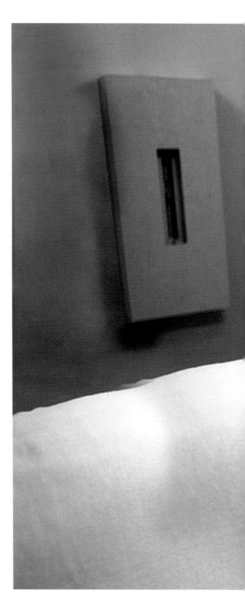

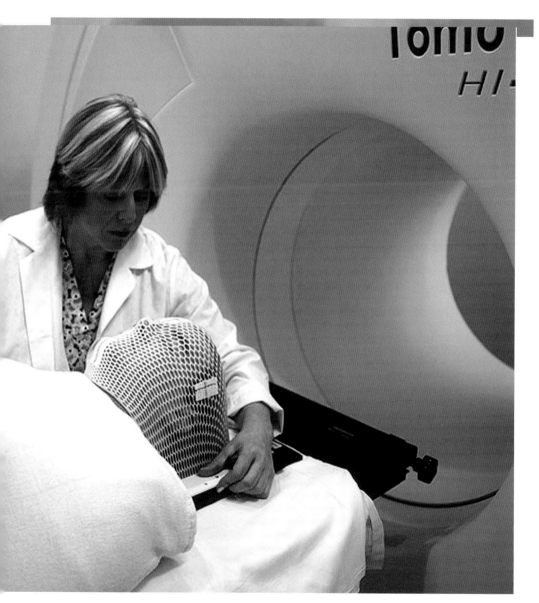

A therapist prepares a cancer patient for radiation treatment. The type of therapy being used here is called TomoTherapy, which enables oncologists to deliver radiation exactly to the tumors instead of affecting normal tissues and organs.

any remaining cancer cells that cannot be seen or in cases where a complete surgical removal was not possible.

In the past, a large or deeply buried tumor in an arm or leg meant amputation of part or all of the affected limb. Modern operating skills allow physicians to opt for limb-sparing surgery in the majority of these cases. Radiation therapy or chemotherapy may be given first to shrink the tumor as much as possible prior to a surgical resection. Moreover, surgeons may be able to replace lost tissue by rebuilding it with a graft from the healthy portions of a patient's body, a metal prosthesis (artificial replacement of a body part), or even a graft from another person's tissues.

Extremely large or aggressive soft tissue sarcomas of the arms and legs may still require the most serious surgeries—amputation and/or removal of all lymph nodes infiltrated by invading cancer cells—to give the patient the best hope for survival.

An Energized Approach

Radiation therapy uses high-energy X-rays or other forms of radiation such as gamma rays to kill cancer cells or keep them from growing. There are several types of radiation therapy used in treating soft tissue sarcomas. External beam radiation therapy is the most common and uses a machine outside the body to send X-rays toward the cancer. With internal radiation therapy, also known as a radiation implant or brachytherapy, a radioactive substance ("seed") is surgically placed into or right next to a tumor to give a more continuous dose of radiation to the tumor(s).

Side effects from radiation therapy depend on the part of the body being treated and the total dose of radiation given. Everyone reacts differently. Radiation therapy itself does not hurt. During treatment, though, a patient may experience one or more of the following: tiredness, tender skin and redness, nausea, diarrhea, sore throat, and hair loss. Usually, these problems disappear fairly quickly after the therapy is finished.

MEDICINE WITH A MISSION

A third method for treating soft tissue sarcomas is chemotherapy, the use of anticancer drugs. Most commonly given orally or injected into the body, these medications travel through the bloodstream to reach their targets. They work by aiming for cells that rapidly or continuously divide as tumor cells do when they are growing.

Unfortunately, what gives chemotherapy agents their power also makes them dangerous. Their attraction to rapidly dividing cells also causes them to attack tissues that also normally divide rapidly. Examples include the bone marrow that supplies the blood-forming cells and disease-fighting cells of the immune system, the linings of the stomach and intestines that take in nutrients from food, the organs of the reproductive system, and the hair follicles. Therefore, patients undergoing chemotherapy must be carefully monitored so that any side effects from the loss of normal cells can be addressed as part of their treatment program.

In many cases, one drug is not enough to completely tackle a soft tissue sarcoma. A combination of chemotherapy agents is usually given to attack the cancer from many angles. The oncologist's treatment plan may also team chemotherapy with surgery and/or radiation therapy for a greater chance of success.

WHEN SHOULD A CLINICAL TRIAL BE CONSIDERED?

For some patients, participating in a clinical trial may be the best course of treatment for their soft tissue sarcoma. Clinical trials are studies conducted by research hospitals and institutions to determine if promising

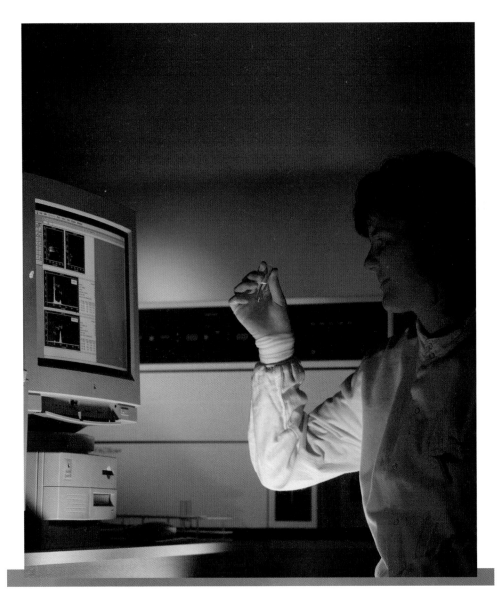

A researcher holds a sample of an anticancer drug while looking at a computer screen. The screen displays data that shows the drug's effectiveness at blocking tumor growth.

experimental therapies are safe and effective and, most important, if they are improvements over traditional cancer treatments.

Patients choose to participate in clinical trials in order to take a more active role in their own health care. They also can gain access to new research treatments before they are widely available and help others by contributing to medical research. Many times, clinical trial patients are those for whom conventional therapies have not been successful; who have recurrence of the cancer after completing treatment; or whose tumors cannot be addressed with standard surgery, radiation, or chemotherapy. There are four major types of clinical trials, classified as phases, which investigate new drugs and treatments at different stages of their development. It is important to know that any treatment used in clinical trials has been extensively tested in the laboratory before being given to humans.

- **In Phase I trials,** researchers test an experimental drug or treatment in a small group of people (usually twenty to eighty) for the first time to evaluate its safety, determine a safe dosage range, and identify side effects.
- **In Phase II trials,** the experimental drug or treatment is given to a larger group of people (one hundred to three hundred) to see if it is effective and to further evaluate its safety.
- **In Phase III trials,** the experimental drug or treatment is given to large groups of people (one thousand to three thousand) to confirm its effectiveness, monitor side effects, compare it to commonly used treatments, and collect information that will allow the experimental drug or treatment to be used safely.
- **In Phase IV trials,** studies are conducted after a drug or treatment enters clinical practice to gather additional information on its risks, benefits, and optimal use.

A patient's personal physician and oncologist will work with the clinical trial team to carefully monitor his or her progress. The patient or doctors can elect to remove the patient at any time during the treatment period. Patients should understand that clinical trials are not without some risks—including the possibility that the experimental drug or treatment may not be effective against the cancer or that it will cause bad side effects.

Before agreeing to participate in a clinical trial, patients should know as much as possible about it. Patients should ask members of the health care team any questions they might have about the study.

There are many resources available for patients to assist them in locating an appropriate clinical trial. These include local hospitals and cancer centers, support groups, and Web sites such as ClinicalTrials.gov, Cancer411.com, and CancerTrialsHelp.org (see also the For More Information section in this book).

WHAT HAPPENS AFTER THERAPY?

Whether a patient undergoes standard treatment for a soft tissue sarcoma or participates in a clinical trial, it is important that he or she continues to receive proper care once the therapy is completed. This care should involve regular medical checkups to monitor the patient's progress following treatment and check for recurrence (the return of cancer in the primary site) or metastasis (the spread of cancer to another part of the body).

The frequency and nature of follow-up care is individualized based on the type of cancer, the type of treatment received, and the person's overall health, including possible treatment-related problems. In general, patients are seen very frequently (about every three months) during the first few years following completion of treatment to monitor for side effects and tumor recurrence, then a little less frequently during later years (once or twice per year).

WAYS TO COPE WITH CANCER

Having cancer is perhaps the greatest challenge a person can face in his or her life. Thankfully, no one has to face that journey alone. There are many forms of help available to see a patient through every stage: diagnosis, treatment, follow-up, and survivorship. Here are just a few:

Support groups: These groups allow patients to meet others with cancer and seek strength from their knowledge, experiences, and understanding. Most major cities and cancer hospitals offer support groups that meet on a regular basis. National organizations, such as the American Cancer Society and the National Cancer Institute, can direct patients to nearby support groups, too.

Alternative or complementary therapies: To deal with treatment side effects, overcome depression and anxiety, and keep their minds focused on the positive side of life, many cancer patients turn to alternative or complementary therapies for help. These therapies do not replace the patient's primary cancer treatment; rather, they make the treatments easier to bear. Examples of such therapies include acupuncture, art or music activities, guided imagery, hypnosis, massage, meditation, mind-body exercises (such as qigong, tai chi, and yoga), and relaxation techniques.

Physical activity: Staying physically active during treatment has many positive benefits. For example, regular exercise stimulates the release of hormones known as endorphins that elevate mood and relieve fatigue. Patients should work with their physicians as to the level, duration, and frequency of physical activity that will work best in their personal situation.

Journaling: Some cancer patients find keeping a journal of their treatment experience to be valuable. Such records can also provide the patient with an opportunity to note personal feelings and thoughts about what he or she is going through. Journals can be kept private like a diary or shared with family, friends, and even strangers.

Blogging: Social media sites such as Facebook, Twitter, and YouTube have given cancer patients a unique way to express their feelings, share their experiences, and find support from the millions worldwide connected by the Internet. Others use blogs and their personal stories to raise public awareness of cancer and seek funding for research.

At these follow-up meetings, the physician or oncologist will likely order blood tests and imaging studies such as CT scans or X-rays to check for sarcoma recurrence and screen for other types of cancers. These tests may or may not be the same ones used to originally diagnose the patient's soft tissue sarcoma.

It is important for patients to keep an updated copy of their cancer treatment records throughout the posttreatment period. Patients may not always see the same doctor for their follow-up care, so having this information available to share with another practitioner can be helpful.

Once a patient has gone five years past treatment without a recurrence or metastasis of the soft tissue sarcoma, he or she is considered in remission (free of cancer). However, cancer screening should continue to be a part of the person's annual medical checkup, as some cancers rarely do come back after five years. People with strong family histories of cancer or known gene mutations linked to cancer syndromes should continue to be screened closely throughout their lifetimes.

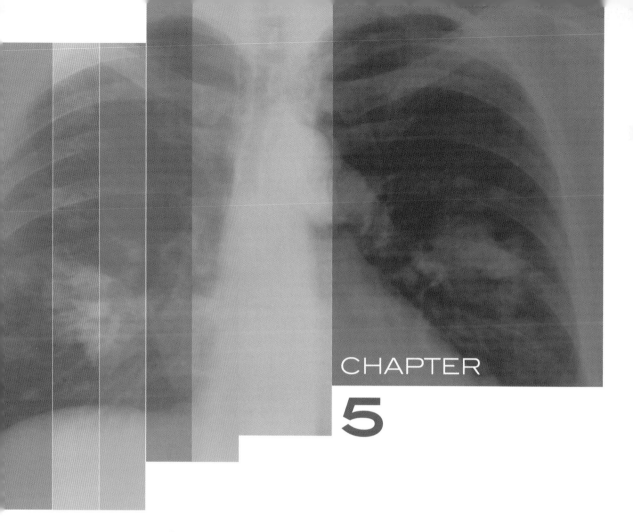

NEW HORIZONS, NEW HOPE

Fifty-fifty. For a patient in 1970 with a soft tissue sarcoma of the arm or leg, those were the odds that the limb would have to be amputated. Even if the surgery was successful, the cancer returned in a third of the cases. Just forty years later, that number has dropped to less than 10 percent for both. The dramatic difference in these odds has been the result of forward-thinking, cutting-edge medical research and clinical trials. Such advancements resulted in PET scans that could potentially detect tumors at earlier states, better radiation treatments, combination drug therapies that attack tumors with

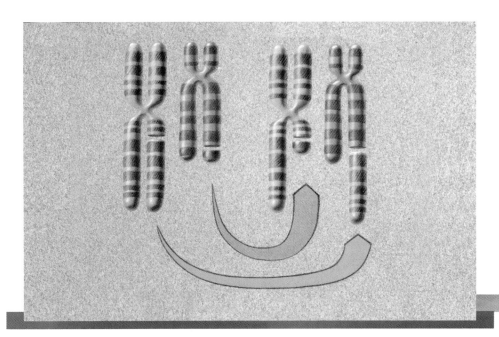

This illustration depicts a genetic mutation resulting from translocation, the switching of part of one chromosome with a piece of another. Translocation may cause some cancers.

different strategies, and improved surgical techniques such as limb preservation strategies.

The same drive to refine, test, and implement improved detection methods and treatments for soft tissue sarcomas continues today. Medical professionals are working at institutions around the globe on innovative research to:

- Explore the origins of sarcomas at the genetic level
- Test new drugs aimed at slowing or halting the progress of sarcomas
- Develop better treatment strategies with available drugs
- Find ways to help the body's immune system subdue sarcoma cancer cells

FOUR TIPS TO A BETTER LIFE FOR CANCER SURVIVORS

Advances in the diagnosis and treatment of soft tissue sarcomas mean that the number of persons who survive the disease grows significantly each year. Following therapy, survivors commonly find themselves switching their focus from how to beat cancer to how to resume a normal life without it. Here are some suggestions to make the transition easier:

Eat well: Choose healthy foods, especially those shown to lessen the risk of cancer, including fruits, fibrous grains, leafy vegetables, and low-fat meats (such as turkey). Achieve and maintain a proper weight for your age, height, and physical condition.

Stay active: If someone enjoyed sports, cooking, or gardening before cancer, there is no reason why that should change after the tumor is out of the picture. Survivors should discuss the conditions and limitations of resuming favorite activities following therapy, especially exercise, with their physician.

Take some chances: Survivors often feel that they've been given a second chance at life and find it easier to take risks and seize the moment. That's not to say a person should take up skydiving or car racing after overcoming cancer; rather, it should be an opportunity to get the most out of his or her life.

Maintain a strong support system: Just because the cancer is gone, a survivor doesn't have to stop reaching out to the friends, relatives, and colleagues who helped him or her beat the disease. Keep in touch and celebrate the victory over cancer together.

Such research can make—and has already made—a difference. Successful cancer treatment in the twenty-first century is the direct result of decades of laboratory and clinical research progress.

GETTING DOWN TO BASICS

In recent years, researchers have made great progress in understanding how certain changes in the genes of soft tissue cells cause sarcomas to develop. For example, studies in Europe and the United States have shown that most patients with synovial tissue sarcomas have a specific translocation between two chromosomes, which contain the genetic material of the cell. A translocation is when one piece of a chromosome somehow breaks off and joins a different chromosome, resulting in the putting together of genes that aren't normally side by side. The impact of this genetic switching is akin to moving the goalie of a hockey team into a forward's spot and putting the forward in front of the goal. Such a "translocation" would certainly result in a breakdown of order, with the out-of-position goalie unlikely to score while the opposing team tallied repeatedly against a player with no experience as a netminder. Translocation

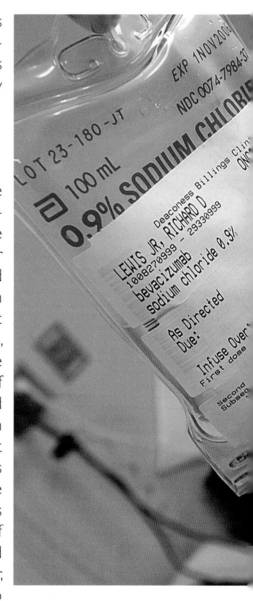

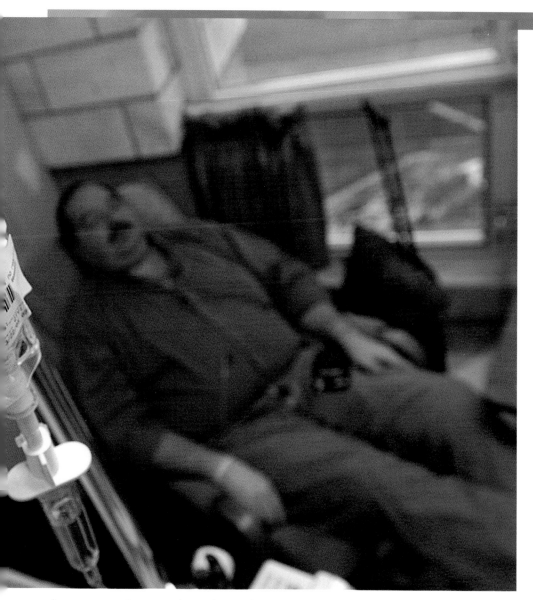

A cancer patient receives chemotherapy treatment with the antiangiogenesis (prevents the formation of blood vessels) drug called bevacizumab. Currently, the effectiveness of bevacizumab, used in combination with other drugs in treating soft tissue sarcomas, is being tested and studied in clinical trials.

between chromosomes in a synovial cell is just as disastrous. Switching parts of the two genes causes their coded instructions to be misread, changing the production of important cell growth and regulation proteins. The result is unchecked growth that produces a tumor.

Knowing what goes wrong with genes related to cancer is important because it often translates into new and improved treatments. Take an innovative treatment known as targeted therapies, for example. These are drugs that specifically block small molecules within cells that are linked to cancers. In the case of a gastrointestinal stromal tumor (GIST), a soft tissue sarcoma of the stomach and intestines, scientists doing genetic studies discovered that a protein called CD117, or c-Kit, normally signals cells in the GI tract to divide and multiply. However, when the gene producing c-Kit is mutated, a bad protein results that allows for rapid, uncontrolled cell growth. This knowledge led medical researchers to look for chemotherapy agents that could block the wayward growth signal from doing its damage. One drug that they found, imatinib (Gleevec), is now standard therapy for treating GISTs that recur after the first tumor is removed.

Hunting for New Remedies

Another experimental therapy for soft tissue sarcomas involves the use of antiangiogenesis drugs. These are medications that block the formation of new blood vessels in tissues. Because tumors grow more rapidly than normal cells, they require more blood to keep them nourished. For example, an antiangiogenesis drug called bevacizumab has been shown to be effective against some sarcomas when given in combination with the chemotherapy drug doxorubicin.

In the war against soft tissue sarcomas, even old enemies among drugs are now being recast as heroes. Thalidomide was taken by thousands of pregnant women worldwide in the late 1950s and early 1960s to relieve morning sickness. Unfortunately, it also resulted in a large

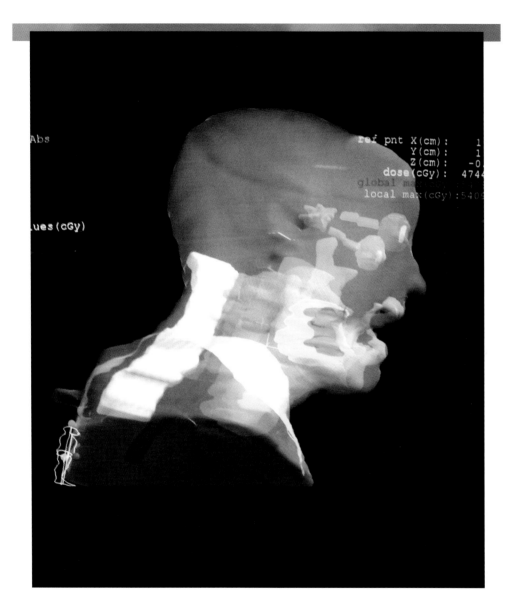

This image shows a patient with head and neck cancer undergoing intensity modulated radiation therapy (IMRT). IMRT uses 3-D computer scans to precisely target tumors with high-intensity doses of radiation while sparing normal tissues.

number of babies being born with missing or shortened limbs and other defects. The comeback for the banned substance began in 1998, when laboratory tests showed it blocked blood vessel formation in leprosy cells. Other researchers suggested thalidomide as a treatment for cancers. Today, clinical trials are under way to define the drug's tumor-fighting potential.

Sometimes Mother Nature, anywhere from the rainforests to the oceans, may be a source for new drugs against soft tissue sarcoma. An ongoing program at the National Cancer Institute to screen plant and marine organisms for cancer-killing materials has yielded a number of potential antitumor agents. One chemical compound discovered through this effort, trabectedin, was extracted in 1984 from sea squirts captured among the coral reefs of the West Indies.

However, isolating enough trabectedin for laboratory and clinical studies wasn't easy. Researchers found that it took about one ton of sea squirts to produce one gram of trabectedin (one teaspoon is approximately four grams). About five grams are necessary to conduct a clinical trial. Fortunately, chemists at Harvard University have developed a means of synthetically manufacturing trabectedin to yield reliable quantities sufficient for study. The drug is currently undergoing Phase II clinical trial testing and proving valuable as a treatment for a variety of pediatric sarcomas.

New Ways to Radiate Hope

Scientific studies and clinical trials are also uncovering better methods to irradiate tumors. One adaptation of traditional external beam radiation that has proved extremely effective for a variety of soft tissue sarcomas is intensity-modulated radiation therapy, or IMRT. The technique uses a sophisticated computer-guided device to safely deliver much higher doses of radiation to a tumor than traditional radiation therapy, while sparing the normal surrounding tissues. IMRT has become the standard radiation therapy used to treat soft tissue sarcomas because it reduces the risk of exposing bones to radiation, thereby reducing the risk of fractures after treatment and allowing more normal bone growth in children and teens.

While IMRT can be used to treat most soft tissue sarcomas in the body, the technique is most beneficial when protecting critical organs, such as the liver, from radiation exposure. Another plus for IMRT is that it effectively distributes radiation throughout a large treatment area, which works well when tumors are deep within thick tissues.

Advancing radiation therapy one step further is a newer form of IMRT known as image-guided radiation therapy, or IGRT. In this procedure, radiation oncologists use imaging devices such as CT scans and MRIs to pinpoint the exact location of a soft tissue sarcoma prior to the delivery of radiotherapy or even during a treatment. This technique helps reduce the amount of healthy tissue exposed to radiation to 0.2 inch (5 millimeters) and, in certain cases, to as little as 0.04 inch (1 mm).

IGRT is particularly useful when a sarcoma is located extremely close to critical areas of the body, such as the spinal column or a major blood vessel. Damage to these critical tissues from excess radiation exposure would be very dangerous, even life-threatening.

PUSHING THE ENVELOPE

Along with advancing the "big three" forms of treatment for soft tissue sarcomas—surgery, radiation, and chemotherapy—and posttherapy options, investigators are exploring a number of promising techniques for certain situations. Among these are the following:

- **Immunotherapy:** This technique uses whole tumor cells or parts of cells (such as proteins on the tumor surface) to stimulate the patient's immune system against his or her specific cancer. It can almost be considered a "personalized" therapy.

Immunotherapy is sort of like getting a vaccination; its goal is to stimulate the immune system to attack foreign invaders or, in this case, tumor cells.

— **Stem cell transplantation:** Because intense chemotherapy often destroys hematopoietic stem cells (immature tissues that develop into red and white blood cells) along with tumor cells, stem cells are harvested and banked from the patient prior to therapy and then used to replenish what is lost.

— **Regional hyperthermia:** With this therapy, electromagnetic energy is used to apply heat (between 104 and 109 degrees Fahrenheit, or 40 to 43 degrees Celsius) to soft tissues in and around tumors at the same time that chemotherapy is given. This method is thought to directly kill cancer cells and increase the flow of blood and oxygen to the area, which can make the tumor more sensitive to drug treatments.

Current chemotherapy, radiation, and surgical treatments for soft tissue sarcomas have increased the five-year survival rates dramatically, even as high as 90 percent for some tumors that are diagnosed at earlier stages (that is, not metastatic) and have lower grades. While that statistic is impressive, much research still needs to be done to better understand soft tissue sarcomas and continue to improve cure rates. Hopefully, the efforts of dedicated researchers and oncologists over the next few years will result in better treatments with fewer side effects, better quality of life for survivors, and even the means to prevent soft tissue sarcomas altogether in the future.

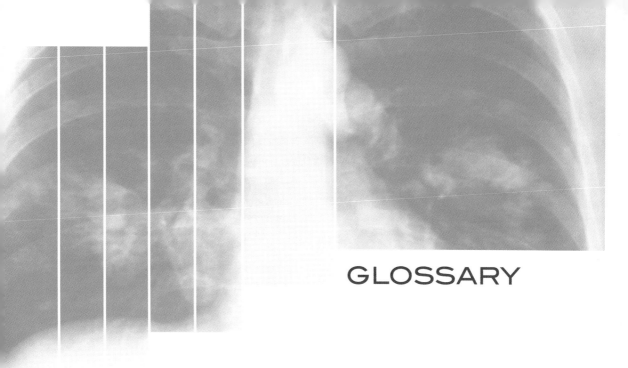

GLOSSARY

abnormally Unusually or unexpectedly; behaving in a way that causes alarm or is undesirable.

aggressive Growing, developing, or spreading quickly.

benign Noncancerous.

biopsy The removal of cells or tissues for examination under the microscope.

cell The basic functional unit of all living organisms; cells are specialized to carry out a specific job, such as a red blood cell that transports oxygen.

chromosome A single piece of coiled DNA containing many genes.

clinical trial Testing of an experimental medicine.

diagnosis Identifying or determining the nature and cause of a disease.

fascia The continuous web of soft tissue found throughout an individual's body.

gene A section of a chromosome with a complete code for producing a specific protein.

grade Assigning a level of abnormality to the cells of a tumor.

hormone A chemical produced in the body that affects the functioning of the body.

hyperthermia The use of heat just above normal body temperature to treat cancer.

incidence The occurrence, rate, or frequency of a disease.

irradiate To treat a tumor by exposing it to radiation waves.

Li-Fraumeni syndrome A rare genetic disorder that generally increases the risk of developing several types of cancer, particularly in children and young adults. It is caused by mutations in the *TP53* gene.

lymph node Any of the small structures located along the circulatory system that filter bacteria and foreign particles from the body.

malignancy A mass of rapidly growing, abnormal cells diagnosed as cancer. Malignant tumors have the potential to spread to other parts of the body (metastasize).

metastasis The spread of a cancer from its point of origin to other parts of the body.

morbidly Having the nature or characteristic of disease.

mutation A change or alteration in the code carried by a gene.

oncologist A doctor who treats cancer.

organ A group of tissues that work together as a single unit.

pathologist A physician who specializes in examining tissues under the microscope and performing laboratory studies to determine the causes of illness or death.

recurrence The return of a cancer that had been successfully treated in the past.

resection The surgical removal of part of an organ.

sarcoma A malignant tumor that develops in the bone or soft tissues of the body.

staging Defining a malignant tumor according to its size and depth, whether or not it has spread to the lymph nodes or to other organs.

stem cell Primitive, unspecialized cells that, under certain conditions, can be transformed into more mature cells with specific functions.

system A group of organs linked together. For example, the major organs of the digestive system are the mouth, esophagus, stomach, and small and large intestines.

tissue A group of similar cells working together. There are four basic types of tissue: muscle, nerve, epidermal (skin), and connective.

translocation A genetic mutation where DNA from one chromosome somehow gets switched to another.

tumor An abnormal mass of cells.

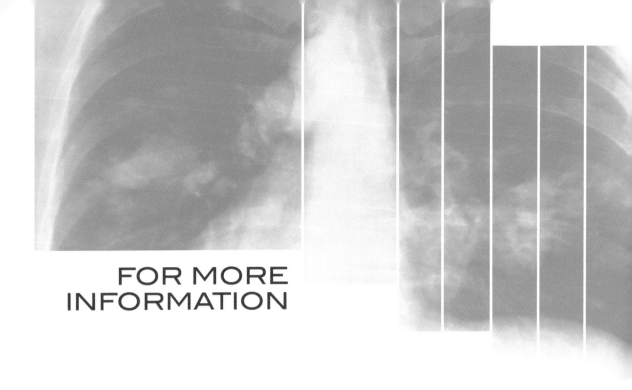

FOR MORE
INFORMATION

American Cancer Society (ACS)
National Cancer Information Center
1599 Clifton Road NE
Atlanta, GA 30329
(800) ACS-2345 (227-2345)
Web site: http://www.cancer.org
The ACS is a nationwide, community-based, voluntary health organization
   dedicated to eliminating cancer as a major health problem by pre-
   venting cancer, saving lives, and diminishing suffering from cancer
   through research, education, advocacy, and service.

American Institute of Cancer Research (AICR)
1759 R Street NW
Washington, DC 20009
(800) 843-8114
Web site: http://www.aicr.org
The AICR helps people make choices that reduce their chances of
   developing cancer. Its mission includes funding research on the rela-

tionship of nutrition, physical activity, and weight management to cancer risk; interpreting the accumulated scientific literature in the field; and educating people on ways to reduce their chances of developing cancer.

Canadian Cancer Society (CCS)
National Office
Suite 200, 10 Alcorn Avenue
Toronto, ON M4V 3B1
Canada
(416) 961-7223
Web site: http://www.cancer.ca
The CCS is a national community-based organization of volunteers whose mission is the eradication of cancer and the enhancement of the quality of life of people living with cancer.

Children's Oncology Group
National Childhood Cancer Foundation
4600 East-West Highway, Suite 600
Bethesda, MD 20814
(800) 458-6223
Web site: http://www.curesearch.org
The Children's Oncology Group is a network of more than five thousand physicians, nurses, and scientists whose collaboration, research, and care have turned childhood cancer from a virtually incurable disease to one with an overall 78 percent cure rate.

Institute of Cancer Research (ICR)
160 Elgin Street, 9th Floor
Address Locator 4809A
Ottawa, ON K1A 0W9

Canada
(888) 603-4178
Web site: http://www.cihr-irsc.gc.ca/e/12506.html
The ICR is one of the thirteen virtual institutes that make up the
Canadian Institutes of Health Research. It is dedicated to supporting
research that reduces the burden of cancer on individuals and families.

Liddy Shriver Sarcoma Initiative
Sarcoma Learning Center
17 Bethea Drive
Ossining, NY 10562
(914) 762-3251
Web site: http://www.sarcomahelp.org/sarcoma.html
The Liddy Shriver Sarcoma Initiative seeks to improve the quality of
life for people dealing with sarcoma. The initiative increases global
public awareness of sarcoma, raises funds to award research grants,
and provides support and timely information to sarcoma patients,
their families, and medical professionals.

National Cancer Institute (NCI)
Cancer Information Service
6116 Executive Boulevard, Room 3036A
Bethesda, MD 20892
(800) 4-CANCER (422-6237)
Web site: http://www.cancer.gov
The NCI, part of the National Institutes of Health, is the U.S. government's principal agency for cancer research and training. It
coordinates the National Cancer Program, which conducts and supports research, training, health information dissemination, and other
programs with respect to the cause, diagnosis, prevention, and treatment of cancer, rehabilitation from cancer, and the continuing care

of cancer patients and the families of cancer patients. For online chats, check out https://cissecure.nci.nih.gov/livehelp/welcome.asp.

Sarcoma Alliance
775 East Blithedale, #334
Mill Valley, CA 94941
(415) 381-7236
Web site: http://www.sarcomaalliance.com
The Sarcoma Alliance strives to extend and improve the lives of sarcoma patients through accurate diagnosis, improved access to care, education, and support.

Sarcoma Foundation of America (SFA)
9884 Main Street
Damascus, MD 20872
(301) 253-8687
Web site: http://www.curesarcoma.org
The SFA advocates for increased research to find new and better therapies with which to treat patients with sarcoma. The foundation is currently establishing chapters in all fifty states.

WEB SITES

Due to the changing nature of Internet links, Rosen Publishing has developed an online list of Web sites related to the subject of this book. This site is updated regularly. Please use this link to access the list:

http://www.rosenlinks.com/cms/sarc

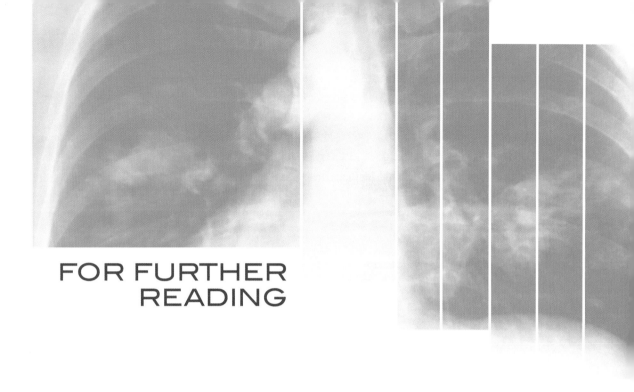

FOR FURTHER READING

Anderson, Greg. *Cancer: 50 Essential Things to Do*. New York, NY: Plume (Penguin Group), 2009.

Barr, Ronald D., et al. *Childhood Cancer: Information for the Patient and Family*. Hamilton, ON, Canada: B. C. Decker, 2001.

Bozzone, Donna M. *Causes of Cancer* (The Biology of Cancer). New York, NY: Chelsea House, 2007

Grealy, Lucy. *Autobiography of a Face*. New York, NY: Harper Perennial, 2003.

Kenny, Paraic A. *Stages of Cancer Development* (The Biology of Cancer). New York, NY: Chelsea House, 2007.

Lyons, Lymna. *Diagnosis and Treatment of Cancer* (The Biology of Cancer). New York, NY: Chelsea House, 2007.

McKinnell, Robert G. *Prevention of Cancer* (The Biology of Cancer). New York, NY: Chelsea House, 2008.

Mooney, Belinda. *Cancer* (At Issue). Farmington Hills, MI: Greenhaven Press, 2007.

Parker, James N., and Philip M. Parker, eds. *The Official Parent's Sourcebook on Childhood Soft Tissue Sarcoma: A Revised and Updated Directory for the Internet Age*. San Diego, CA: ICON Health Publications, 2002.

Pollock, Raphael E. *Soft Tissue Sarcomas* (American Cancer Society Atlas of Clinical Oncology). Hamilton, ON, Canada: B. C. Decker, 2002.

Silver, Julie K. *What Helped Get Me Through: Cancer Survivors Share Wisdom and Hope*. Atlanta, GA: American Cancer Society, 2008.

Silverstein, Alvin, et al. *Cancer: Conquering a Deadly Disease*. New York, NY: Twenty-First Century Books, 2004.

Stokes, Angela. *The Monster I Battle: Living with Sarcomas*. Frederick, MD: PublishAmerica, 2005.

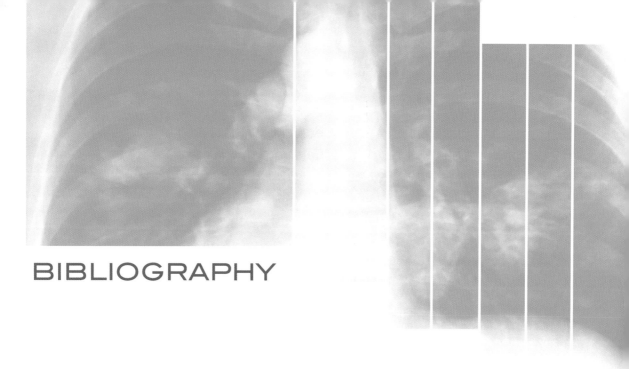

BIBLIOGRAPHY

American Cancer Society. "Rhabdomyosarcoma." Retrieved November 10, 2009 (http://www.cancer.org/docroot/CRI/CRI_0.asp).

American Cancer Society. "Sarcoma—Adult Soft Tissue Cancer." Retrieved November 10, 2009 (http://www.cancer.org/docroot/lrn/lrn_0.asp).

Eyre, Harmon. *Informed Decisions: Second Edition*. Atlanta, GA: American Cancer Society, 2002.

Genetics Home Reference. "Li-Fraumeni Syndrome." Retrieved November 13, 2009 (http://ghr.nlm.nih.gov/condition=lifraumenisyndrome).

MD Anderson Cancer Center. "Soft Tissue Sarcoma." Retrieved November 11, 2009 (http://www.mdanderson.org/patient-and-cancer-information/cancer-information/cancer-types/soft-tissue-sarcoma/index.html)

Medline Plus. "Soft Tissue Sarcoma." Retrieved November 12, 2009 (http://www.nlm.nih.gov/medlineplus/softtissuesarcoma.html).

Memorial Sloan-Kettering Cancer Center. "Soft Tissue Sarcoma." Retrieved November 11, 2009 (http://www.mskcc.org/mskcc/html/435.cfm).

National Cancer Institute. "Cancer Statistics." Retrieved November 10, 2009 (http://www.cancer.gov/statistics).

National Cancer Institute. "Soft Tissue Sarcoma." Retrieved November 10, 2009 (http://www.cancer.gov/cancertopics/factsheet/sites-types/soft-tissue-sarcoma).

Ohio State University Comprehensive Cancer Center. "Soft Tissue Sarcoma." Retrieved November 12, 2009 (http://www.jamesline.com/cancertypes/softtissue/Pages/index.asp).

Pollock, Raphael E. *Soft Tissue Sarcomas* (American Cancer Society Atlas of Clinical Oncology). Hamilton, ON, Canada: B. C. Decker, 2002.

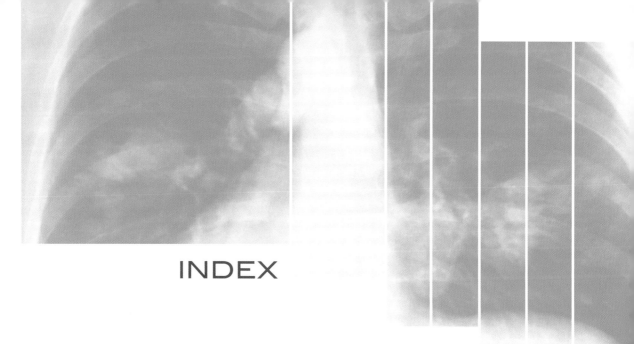

INDEX

ABOUT THE AUTHOR

Michael E. Newman is a broad-based communicator with an extensive and award-winning record in three branches of communications: public relations, journalism, and broadcast media. His thirty-year career has included positions in science and medical communications, corporate and government public affairs, broadcast TV and radio, and mass market publications. He also has been a successful writer for twenty-five years, primarily on medical and science topics. Newman earned a Bachelor of Science degree in microbiology from Clemson University and a Bachelor of Arts degree in communications from the University of Houston. A native of Houston, Texas, Newman currently resides with his family in Derwood, Maryland, outside of Washington, D.C.

PHOTO CREDITS

Cover, p. 1 David Becker/Stone/Getty Images; cover (top), pp. 4–5 (bottom) Punchstock; back cover, pp. 3, 6, 14, 22, 30, 41, 51, 54, 58, 60, 62 National Cancer Institute; p. 5 (top) Stock Montage/Archive Photos/Getty Images; p. 7 LifeART image © (2011) Lippincott Williams & Wilkins. All rights reserved; p. 11 Dorling Kindersley/Getty Images; pp. 12, 31 Science Photo Library/Custom Medical Stock Photo; p. 15 Jonathan Alcorn/Zuma Press; pp. 17, 32–33, 42 National Cancer Institute; p. 19 AFP/Getty Images; p. 24 CNRI/Photo Researchers, Inc.; p. 27 Dr. P. Marazzi/Photo Researchers, Inc.; p. 36 Colin Cuthbert/Science Photo Library/Custom Medical Stock Photo; pp. 44–45 © AP Images; p. 47 Custom Medical Stock Photo.

Designer: Evelyn Horovicz; Editor: Kathy Kuhtz Campbell; Photo Researcher: Peter Tomlinson